Managing Fibromyalgia

A Comprehensive Self-Care Plan

Proven Strategies to Alleviate Pain, Combat Fatigue, and Improve Quality of Life

Graham Julian Oliver

Disclaimer

The information provided in *Managing Fibromyalgia: A Comprehensive Self-Care Plan* is intended for general informational purposes only and is not a substitute for professional medical advice, diagnosis, or treatment. The author and publisher are not licensed medical professionals and do not provide medical services. Always seek the advice of your physician or another qualified health provider with any questions you may have regarding a medical condition or treatment.

While the strategies and information shared in this book may help manage symptoms of fibromyalgia and chronic pain, individual results may vary. It is essential to evaluate your circumstances and consult with a healthcare professional before implementing any changes to your treatment plan or self-care routine.

The author and publisher do not endorse or assume any responsibility for any individual, product, website, organization, or other names that may be referenced or mentioned in this book. Any mention of such entities is for informational purposes only and should not be construed as an endorsement.

By using this book, you acknowledge and agree that you are solely responsible for your health and well-being. The author and publisher shall not be liable for any damages arising from the use or inability to use this book or the information contained herein.

About This Book

Managing Fibromyalgia: A Comprehensive Self-Care Plan provides an essential roadmap for individuals navigating the complex world of chronic pain and fibromyalgia relief. With an empathetic approach, it demystifies the condition, beginning by laying out a clear understanding of fibromyalgia, including its symptoms, prevalence, and the significant impact it can have on daily life. By addressing common misconceptions, this book empowers readers with accurate knowledge, equipping them to advocate for their own care and make informed decisions alongside healthcare providers.

Self-care is presented as a fundamental aspect of managing fibromyalgia effectively, enabling readers to create personalized strategies for long-term relief. The book introduces a multi-faceted approach to pain management, covering an extensive range of therapies from medication to alternative treatments such as acupuncture, massage, and cognitive behavioral therapy (CBT). Readers learn the benefits of heat and cold therapy, the role of diet in reducing inflammation, and the importance of rest and pacing activities, along with practical advice for developing a tailored pain management plan.

Nutrition is highlighted as a cornerstone in managing fibromyalgia symptoms, with guidance on anti-inflammatory foods, supplements like vitamin D and magnesium, and the importance of hydration. The book provides readers with tips on meal planning and tracking food sensitivities, making it easier to incorporate healthy eating habits that may positively impact fatigue, pain, and overall energy levels. This section also advises on budget-friendly ways to prepare balanced meals, making dietary changes more accessible and sustainable.

Exercise and physical activity are crucial elements for individuals with fibromyalgia, yet the book acknowledges the need for gentle, low-impact exercises to avoid overexertion. It offers a well-rounded look at stretching, aerobic exercises, and the calming effects of yoga and tai chi, while emphasizing the importance of listening to one's body. Through motivational strategies and tailored workout suggestions, readers gain confidence in establishing a routine that enhances flexibility, strength, and energy without aggravating symptoms.

Recognizing the importance of restorative sleep, the book delves into sleep disturbances unique to fibromyalgia. From creating a sleep-conducive environment to establishing a bedtime routine, readers are equipped with tools to improve their sleep quality. It also addresses the use of sleep aids, relaxation techniques, and the impact of lifestyle factors such as caffeine on sleep, helping readers develop a holistic approach to rest that significantly enhances their quality of life.

Stress management techniques are another essential focus, as the book highlights the strong connection between stress and symptom flare-ups. Readers are guided through various methods, including breathing exercises, mindfulness, and progressive muscle relaxation, alongside advice on time management, setting boundaries, and finding joy in hobbies and socializing. This comprehensive approach enables readers to identify stress triggers and develop proactive methods to manage them, promoting overall emotional and physical well-being.

A robust support system is emphasized as a critical component in managing fibromyalgia effectively. This guide helps readers understand the value of educating friends and family, finding support groups, and building relationships with healthcare providers who understand their condition. It also explores how community resources and online groups can offer solidarity, encouragement, and practical advice, fostering a network of understanding and empathy.

Lastly, *Managing Fibromyalgia* underscores the importance of tracking progress, as readers learn to monitor symptoms, assess treatment effectiveness, and adjust their self-care strategies as needed. Through journaling, setting realistic goals, and evaluating dietary and lifestyle adjustments, readers develop a flexible approach to symptom management that adapts to their evolving needs. By celebrating small victories and learning from setbacks, readers are empowered to navigate the ups and downs of fibromyalgia with resilience and optimism.

Each section of this guide is crafted to equip individuals with tools, insights, and encouragement for a proactive approach to fibromyalgia, helping them achieve meaningful improvements in their quality of life and maintain hope for a fulfilling future.

Table of Contents

Introduction

Definition of Fibromyalgia and Its Symptoms

Fibromyalgia is a chronic condition characterized by widespread musculoskeletal pain, fatigue, and heightened sensitivity to pain. People with fibromyalgia often experience symptoms such as tender points on the body, stiffness, and cognitive issues, often referred to as "fibro fog." This fog includes difficulties with concentration, memory, and mental clarity. Other symptoms include sleep disturbances, headaches, and sensitivity to noise, lights, or temperature.

Diagnosis can be challenging, as fibromyalgia symptoms overlap with other disorders. However, doctors typically use physical exams, symptom history, and specific criteria, like pain duration and intensity, to diagnose it. Understanding these symptoms helps in forming a comprehensive self-care plan, as well as finding effective treatment options.

Overview of Its Impact on Daily Life

Living with fibromyalgia can deeply affect one's daily routines, energy levels, and emotional well-being. Tasks like getting out of bed, focusing at work, or socializing with friends can become daunting due to chronic pain and fatigue. The unpredictable nature of flare-ups often makes planning challenging, affecting personal, social, and professional areas of life.

This constant struggle can lead to feelings of frustration and isolation, impacting mental health and increasing stress. For many, creating a balanced daily routine, including short rest periods and pacing activities, is crucial. Developing strategies to manage stress, enhance sleep, and balance responsibilities can greatly improve life quality for individuals with fibromyalgia.

Importance of Self-Care

Empowering Individuals to Manage Their Symptoms

To effectively manage fibromyalgia symptoms, it's essential to adopt a mindset of empowerment, focusing on active participation in one's care. Start by setting realistic goals, such as reducing pain by a specific amount each week or gradually increasing activity levels. Regularly track symptoms in a journal or digital app to identify patterns and triggers, as this can offer clarity on what aggravates pain or fatigue. Knowledge is a powerful tool, so educate yourself on the latest management techniques, and seek resources like support groups, where you can learn from others facing similar challenges.

Developing stress management techniques can significantly impact symptom severity. Practices like mindfulness, meditation, and gentle yoga encourage relaxation, which can reduce pain sensitivity and improve sleep. Mindful breathing exercises help calm the nervous system, while progressive muscle relaxation can ease tension in specific muscle groups. By consistently using these techniques, you build resilience against stressors that can worsen fibromyalgia symptoms, making you feel more in control of your health.

Creating a Personalized Approach for Long-Term Relief

Personalized care plans are invaluable for fibromyalgia management, as each person's experience with the condition is unique. Start by working with a healthcare provider to assess your specific symptoms and identify strategies that could offer relief. This might include a combination of medication, physical therapy, and lifestyle adjustments. Tracking how you respond to each intervention over time helps you fine-tune your approach, allowing you to focus on what's most effective for your body.

Integrating a balance of physical activity, diet adjustments, and rest can create a sustainable approach to symptom management. Activities like gentle stretching or low-impact exercises (e.g., swimming or walking) promote flexibility and endurance without overstraining. Prioritize nutrient-rich foods that help reduce inflammation, such as leafy greens, berries, and fatty fish, while limiting inflammatory foods like processed sugars. Together, these adjustments can create a stable foundation for long-term symptom management, giving you more control over your daily well-being.

Empowering Individuals to Manage Their Symptoms

To effectively manage fibromyalgia symptoms, it's essential to adopt a mindset of empowerment, focusing on active participation in one's care. Start by setting realistic goals, such as reducing pain by a specific amount each week or gradually increasing activity levels. Regularly track symptoms in a journal or digital app to identify patterns and triggers, as this can offer clarity on what aggravates pain or fatigue. Knowledge is a powerful tool, so educate yourself on the latest management techniques, and seek resources like support groups, where you can learn from others facing similar challenges.

Developing stress management techniques can significantly impact symptom severity. Practices like mindfulness, meditation, and gentle yoga encourage relaxation, which can reduce pain sensitivity and improve sleep. Mindful breathing exercises help calm the nervous system, while progressive muscle relaxation can ease tension in specific muscle groups. By consistently using these techniques, you build resilience against stressors that can worsen fibromyalgia symptoms, making you feel more in control of your health.

Creating a Personalized Approach for Long-Term Relief

Personalized care plans are invaluable for fibromyalgia management, as each person's experience with the condition is unique. Start by working with a healthcare provider to assess your specific symptoms and identify strategies that could offer relief. This might include a combination of medication, physical therapy, and lifestyle adjustments. Tracking how you respond to each intervention over time helps you fine-tune your approach, allowing you to focus on what's most effective for your body.

Integrating a balance of physical activity, diet adjustments, and rest can create a sustainable approach to symptom management. Activities like gentle stretching or low-impact exercises (e.g., swimming or walking) promote flexibility and endurance without overstraining. Prioritize nutrient-rich foods that help reduce inflammation, such as leafy greens, berries, and fatty fish, while limiting inflammatory foods like processed sugars. Together, these adjustments can create a stable foundation for long-term symptom management, giving you more control over your daily well-being.

CHAPTER 1:

Understanding Fibromyalgia

Explanation of What Fibromyalgia Is

Fibromyalgia is a chronic condition characterized by widespread musculoskeletal pain, fatigue, and tenderness in localized areas. It often affects how the brain processes pain signals, leading to an amplified perception of pain. This disorder can disrupt daily functioning and quality of life, making self-care essential for those living with it.

Understanding fibromyalgia involves recognizing its multifaceted nature, including physical, emotional, and cognitive symptoms. A comprehensive approach to managing fibromyalgia often includes lifestyle modifications, medical treatment, and supportive therapies to alleviate discomfort and enhance well-being.

Symptoms: Pain, Fatigue, Sleep Disturbances

Common symptoms of fibromyalgia include persistent pain, fatigue that does not improve with rest, and sleep disturbances such as insomnia or restless legs. Pain is often described as a constant dull ache, affecting various body parts and sometimes flaring up with physical or emotional stress.

To manage these symptoms, individuals can adopt a combination of pain relief strategies like over-the-counter pain relievers, gentle exercise, and relaxation techniques. Establishing a regular sleep routine, including winding down before bed and creating a comfortable sleep environment, can help mitigate sleep disturbances.

Common Triggers: Stress, Weather, Physical Activity

Fibromyalgia symptoms can be exacerbated by various triggers, including stress, changes in weather, and excessive physical activity. Stress management techniques such as mindfulness, yoga, and deep-breathing exercises can significantly reduce symptom flare-ups.

Additionally, being aware of weather changes, particularly temperature fluctuations and humidity, can help individuals plan their activities and self-care accordingly. Striking a balance between activity and rest is essential for managing fibromyalgia effectively.

The Role of Genetics and Environment

Research suggests that both genetics and environmental factors contribute to the development of fibromyalgia. Family history can increase susceptibility, indicating a genetic link, while environmental triggers such as infections, trauma, or psychological stress may also play a role.

Understanding these influences can empower individuals to identify their unique triggers and customize their self-care strategies. Engaging in regular discussions with healthcare providers about family medical history can also inform personalized management plans.

How Fibromyalgia Is Diagnosed

Diagnosing fibromyalgia typically involves a comprehensive evaluation of symptoms and medical history, as there are no definitive tests for the condition. Healthcare providers often use criteria established by the American College of Rheumatology, which includes widespread pain lasting more than three months and the presence of specific tender points.

To facilitate the diagnosis, patients can keep a symptom diary documenting pain levels, fatigue, and any associated triggers. This information can provide valuable insights for healthcare providers in confirming a fibromyalgia diagnosis and developing an effective management plan.

Difference Between Fibromyalgia and Other Conditions

Fibromyalgia can be confused with other conditions that cause chronic pain, such as chronic fatigue syndrome, rheumatoid arthritis, and lupus. However, fibromyalgia is characterized by widespread pain without joint inflammation, which distinguishes it from these other diseases.

Educating oneself about these differences can aid in better communication with healthcare providers. It is crucial to discuss all symptoms and concerns during medical appointments to ensure an accurate diagnosis and appropriate treatment options.

Prevalence and Demographics Affected

Fibromyalgia affects an estimated 2-8% of the global population, with a higher prevalence in women than men. It commonly manifests in middle-aged adults, although it can occur at any age. Awareness of these demographics can help patients feel less isolated in their experience.

For those affected, connecting with support groups or online communities can provide a sense of belonging and shared understanding. Knowledge of fibromyalgia's prevalence can encourage individuals to advocate for their health and seek necessary care.

Impact on Mental Health and Well-Being

Living with fibromyalgia can significantly impact mental health, leading to issues like depression, anxiety, and decreased quality of life. The chronic nature of pain and fatigue can contribute to feelings of hopelessness or frustration, making emotional support vital.

Incorporating mental health strategies such as therapy, support groups, and mindfulness practices can foster resilience. Individuals should prioritize self-compassion and seek professional help when needed to address mental health concerns alongside their physical symptoms.

Understanding the Neurobiology of Pain

Fibromyalgia involves complex neurobiological mechanisms that alter how the brain and nervous system process pain signals. Research indicates that individuals with fibromyalgia may have heightened sensitivity to pain due to changes in brain chemistry and neurotransmitter function.

To address these neurobiological aspects, treatments such as cognitive behavioral therapy (CBT) and medications that affect neurotransmitters can be beneficial. Understanding these processes can empower individuals to seek appropriate interventions that target both physical and emotional dimensions of pain.

Myths and Misconceptions

There are several myths surrounding fibromyalgia, such as the belief that it is not a real disease or that it is purely a psychological condition. These misconceptions can lead to stigma and misunderstanding, making it essential for individuals to educate themselves and others about fibromyalgia.

Dispelling these myths involves sharing accurate information and personal experiences with fibromyalgia. Engaging in conversations about the condition can help foster understanding and compassion from friends, family, and the broader community.

Importance of a Support System

A robust support system is crucial for individuals managing fibromyalgia, as it can alleviate feelings of isolation and provide emotional and practical assistance. Support may come from family, friends, healthcare providers, or support groups, each offering unique benefits.

To build a supportive network, individuals should communicate openly about their needs and limitations. Participating in support groups, either in-person or online, can help connect with others facing similar challenges and provide a sense of community.

Resources for Information and Support

Numerous resources are available for individuals seeking information and support for fibromyalgia. Reputable organizations, such as the National Fibromyalgia Association, provide educational materials, research updates, and access to support groups.

Additionally, online forums and social media platforms can connect individuals with others who share their experiences. Utilizing these resources can empower individuals to take charge of their health and stay informed about the latest developments in fibromyalgia research and treatment.

Setting Realistic Expectations for Treatment

Managing fibromyalgia often requires a multifaceted approach, and setting realistic expectations for treatment is essential. While some strategies may offer significant relief, others may take time to yield results, and not every method will work for every individual.

Being patient and flexible with treatment plans can foster a sense of control and reduce frustration. It's important to celebrate small victories and to discuss any challenges with healthcare providers to adjust approaches as necessary.

CHAPTER 2:

Pain Management Strategies

Importance of a Multi-Faceted Approach

A multi-faceted approach to managing fibromyalgia recognizes that each individual experiences the condition differently. By combining various strategies—medication, therapy, lifestyle changes, and self-care techniques—patients can find a more effective way to alleviate symptoms. This comprehensive plan ensures that all aspects of health are considered, including physical, emotional, and social factors, promoting a more holistic way of managing the condition.

Implementing this approach means being open to trying different therapies and practices, tracking what works best, and adjusting as needed. By collaborating with healthcare providers, patients can tailor their management plan to their unique needs, optimizing their chances of achieving relief and improving their overall quality of life.

Medication Options: Analgesics, Antidepressants, Anticonvulsants

Medications play a crucial role in managing fibromyalgia symptoms. Analgesics, such as acetaminophen and NSAIDs, can help reduce pain, while antidepressants like duloxetine and milnacipran target both pain and mood issues, which are common in fibromyalgia. Anticonvulsants, such as gabapentin and pregabalin, can also be effective in reducing nerve pain and discomfort.

To find the right medication, it's essential to work closely with a healthcare provider who can assess individual needs and monitor any side effects. Patients should discuss their experiences and symptoms regularly, as adjustments in dosage or medication type may be necessary for optimal pain management.

Non-Pharmacological Therapies: Acupuncture, Massage, and Chiropractic Care

Non-pharmacological therapies offer alternative options for fibromyalgia relief. Acupuncture involves inserting thin needles into specific points on the body to alleviate pain and improve energy flow, providing a relaxing experience that can reduce muscle tension. Massage therapy can relieve stress, improve circulation, and reduce pain by loosening tight muscles and promoting relaxation.

Chiropractic care focuses on spinal alignment and the body's musculoskeletal system, helping to relieve pain and improve function. Regular sessions can enhance mobility and overall well-being, making them valuable components of a comprehensive self-care plan.

Heat and Cold Therapy Techniques

Heat and cold therapy can significantly alleviate fibromyalgia symptoms. Applying heat—through heating pads, warm baths, or heat wraps—can help relax tight muscles and improve blood flow, reducing pain and stiffness. This technique is particularly beneficial during flare-ups or when experiencing muscle soreness.

Conversely, cold therapy, such as ice packs or cold compresses, can numb areas of pain and reduce inflammation. Alternating between heat and cold can be an effective way to manage discomfort and help the body recover after physical activity or during periods of increased pain.

The Role of Physical Therapy

Physical therapy is essential for developing a personalized exercise plan that caters to an individual's capabilities and limitations. A trained physical therapist can guide patients through gentle exercises designed to improve strength, flexibility, and endurance, all crucial for managing fibromyalgia. This approach not only helps alleviate pain but also enhances physical function and mobility.

Incorporating physical therapy into a self-care plan means setting realistic goals and gradually increasing activity levels. Consistency is key; even short sessions of light exercise can lead to significant improvements in overall well-being and pain management.

Mindfulness and Meditation for Pain Relief

Mindfulness and meditation are powerful tools for managing fibromyalgia pain. These practices encourage individuals to focus on the present moment and become more aware of their thoughts and feelings without judgment. Techniques such as guided imagery or deep breathing can help reduce stress and anxiety, which often exacerbate pain levels.

To implement mindfulness, set aside a few minutes daily to practice meditation or mindfulness exercises. Apps or online resources can provide guidance, making it easier for beginners to get started and gradually incorporate these practices into their daily routine.

Cognitive Behavioral Therapy (CBT) Approaches

Cognitive Behavioral Therapy (CBT) helps individuals identify and change negative thought patterns that contribute to pain and stress. By learning to challenge unhelpful beliefs and develop coping strategies, patients can improve their emotional well-being and reduce the impact of fibromyalgia symptoms. CBT often involves structured sessions with a trained therapist who can provide support and guidance.

To apply CBT principles, individuals can start journaling about their thoughts and feelings related to pain. Recognizing patterns and triggers can help them implement coping strategies, ultimately leading to better emotional regulation and pain management.

Importance of Rest and Pacing Activities

Rest and pacing activities are vital for managing fibromyalgia, as overexertion can lead to increased pain and fatigue. Patients should learn to recognize their limits and incorporate regular rest periods throughout their day to recharge. This might mean breaking tasks into smaller, manageable segments and scheduling downtime to prevent burnout.

Establishing a balanced routine that includes both activity and rest is essential. By prioritizing self-care and understanding the importance of pacing, individuals can minimize the risk of flare-ups and maintain a more consistent level of functioning.

The Impact of Diet on Inflammation and Pain

Diet can significantly influence inflammation levels and pain in fibromyalgia. Consuming a balanced diet rich in anti-inflammatory foods—such as fruits, vegetables, whole grains, and healthy fats—can help reduce symptoms. Limiting processed foods, sugars, and trans fats may also alleviate pain and improve overall health.

To implement dietary changes, start by incorporating more whole foods into meals while reducing processed options. Keeping a food diary can help individuals identify any foods that may trigger symptoms and adjust their diet accordingly.

Monitoring Pain Levels with a Pain Diary

Keeping a pain diary is an effective way for individuals to track their pain levels, triggers, and responses to various treatments. Documenting daily pain intensity, activities, mood, and any medications taken can help identify patterns and correlations that are crucial for effective management. This information can also be valuable when consulting with healthcare providers.

To start a pain diary, choose a format—either digital or handwritten—that is easy to use. Regular entries will empower individuals to take control of their pain management and facilitate more informed discussions with their healthcare team.

Collaborating with Healthcare Providers

Effective collaboration with healthcare providers is essential for managing fibromyalgia. Patients should communicate openly about their symptoms, treatment responses, and any concerns they may have. This ongoing dialogue allows providers to tailor treatment plans and make informed recommendations.

Regular check-ins with a primary care physician or specialists, such as rheumatologists or pain management experts, can help ensure that all aspects of care are being addressed. Patients should advocate for themselves and seek second opinions if they feel their concerns are not being taken seriously.

Alternative Therapies: Aromatherapy and Essential Oils

Alternative therapies like aromatherapy can complement traditional treatments for fibromyalgia. Essential oils, such as lavender, eucalyptus, or peppermint, can promote relaxation and relieve stress. Using these oils in diffusers, baths, or through topical applications can enhance overall well-being and help manage pain.

To incorporate aromatherapy into a self-care plan, start by exploring different essential oils and their properties. Experimenting with various applications can help individuals find the scents and methods that work best for them, creating a calming environment that supports pain relief.

Creating a Personalized Pain Management Plan

Developing a personalized pain management plan involves identifying which strategies work best for the individual. This plan should integrate medication, therapies, lifestyle changes, and self-care practices tailored to personal preferences and needs. It's essential to be flexible and willing to adjust the plan as symptoms change.

To create this plan, patients can consult with healthcare providers to establish clear goals and strategies. Regularly reviewing and modifying the plan based on experiences and outcomes will lead to more effective pain management and improved quality of life.

CHAPTER 3:

Nutrition and Fibromyalgia

The Connection between Diet and Fibromyalgia Symptoms

Diet plays a crucial role in managing fibromyalgia symptoms, as certain foods can either alleviate or exacerbate pain, fatigue, and other related issues. For instance, a diet high in whole foods, vegetables, lean proteins, and healthy fats can help regulate inflammation levels and support overall body function. People with fibromyalgia may experience less pain and discomfort when they avoid foods that commonly trigger inflammation, such as refined sugars, fried foods, and processed snacks.

Understanding the impact of diet on fibromyalgia symptoms also means noting any personal sensitivities to specific foods, like gluten or dairy, which can intensify discomfort. Testing various foods and observing reactions is a helpful way to customize a diet that minimizes symptoms. Over time, a mindful approach to eating can empower individuals with fibromyalgia to experience improved energy and manage symptoms more effectively.

Anti-Inflammatory Foods to Consider

Incorporating anti-inflammatory foods can be a powerful way to support fibromyalgia management. Foods like leafy greens (spinach, kale), fatty fish (salmon, sardines), nuts, seeds, and berries are rich in antioxidants and omega-3 fatty acids that help reduce inflammation. These nutrients not only support joint and muscle health but also may alleviate chronic pain associated with fibromyalgia.

Adding spices such as turmeric and ginger can further enhance the anti-inflammatory effects, as they contain compounds that block inflammatory pathways in the body. Including a variety of these foods regularly helps in building a nutrient-dense, pain-relieving diet that addresses inflammation from multiple angles, potentially leading to noticeable improvements in symptoms.

Foods to Avoid: Processed Foods, Sugars, and Gluten

Avoiding processed foods, excess sugars, and gluten is often beneficial for people with fibromyalgia. Processed foods, which often contain additives, preservatives, and unhealthy fats, can trigger inflammation, increase fatigue, and worsen fibromyalgia pain. Sugary foods, especially those with high-fructose corn syrup, can lead to blood sugar fluctuations, contributing to energy crashes and aggravating symptoms.

Additionally, some individuals with fibromyalgia may have sensitivities to gluten, which could cause additional digestive issues and inflammation. Steering clear of these foods and opting for whole, natural options—like fresh vegetables, fruits, and lean proteins—can help reduce symptom flare-ups and support consistent energy levels.

Importance of Hydration

Hydration is key to fibromyalgia management, as staying well-hydrated can reduce fatigue, improve muscle function, and support joint lubrication. Drinking enough water daily—typically around eight 8-ounce glasses—helps to flush out toxins and reduce inflammation, which can significantly impact pain levels. Mild dehydration can worsen muscle cramps, brain fog, and overall fatigue, common symptoms in fibromyalgia.

In addition to plain water, herbal teas and electrolyte-rich options like coconut water can contribute to hydration. Avoiding excessive caffeine and sugary beverages, which can dehydrate the body, is equally important. By prioritizing hydration, individuals can experience a clearer mind, better mobility, and enhanced symptom control.

The Role of Supplements: Vitamin D, Magnesium, Omega-3s

Supplements can provide essential nutrients that may help alleviate fibromyalgia symptoms, particularly when certain deficiencies exist. Vitamin D supports immune function and bone health, and research suggests it may reduce pain sensitivity. Magnesium, known for its muscle-relaxing properties, can help ease muscle stiffness and cramps, common in fibromyalgia.

Omega-3 fatty acids, found in fish oil, reduce inflammation and may positively impact both pain and mood. Always consult with a healthcare provider before starting supplements, as they can recommend appropriate dosages and identify any possible interactions. Supplements, combined with a nutrient-rich diet, can support comprehensive symptom management.

Meal Planning for Convenience and Health

Meal planning can simplify healthy eating for fibromyalgia sufferers by reducing the effort and stress involved in preparing nutritious meals. Preparing meals in advance, such as cooking a batch of quinoa or chopping vegetables for the week, can save time and energy. Focus on easy-to-make dishes that include anti-inflammatory ingredients like leafy greens, lean proteins, and healthy fats.

Additionally, keeping nutritious snacks handy, like nuts or yogurt, can help maintain energy levels throughout the day. Planning balanced, anti-inflammatory meals that align with personal food tolerances can improve consistency in diet and symptom management, making it easier to avoid triggers and maintain a pain-reducing lifestyle.

Importance of Regular Meal Schedules

Eating on a regular schedule supports blood sugar balance and helps maintain consistent energy levels, which is essential for managing fibromyalgia symptoms. Skipping meals can lead to low energy, irritability, and increased fatigue. Aim for balanced meals and snacks at consistent times to help the body maintain stable energy.

Regular meal timing also allows the body to anticipate and better manage nutritional intake, preventing spikes in fatigue or discomfort. Consistent meal patterns make it easier to track symptom triggers and manage energy, helping to stabilize both mood and pain levels throughout the day.

The Benefits of Antioxidants

Antioxidants combat oxidative stress in the body, which can worsen pain and fatigue associated with fibromyalgia. Including foods rich in antioxidants, such as berries, dark chocolate, and nuts, helps reduce cell damage and inflammation. These foods contain vitamins C and E, selenium, and flavonoids that protect cells and promote overall wellness.

In addition to dietary sources, antioxidants can be found in supplements, but whole food sources tend to offer the best absorption and additional health benefits. Regularly consuming antioxidant-rich foods can support immune function and potentially reduce the frequency and intensity of fibromyalgia flare-ups.

Foods That May Help Improve Sleep Quality

Certain foods may promote better sleep, which is vital for individuals with fibromyalgia as poor sleep can exacerbate symptoms. Foods like cherries, almonds, and warm milk contain nutrients that support melatonin production and relaxation, helping improve sleep quality and duration.

Complex carbohydrates, such as sweet potatoes or oatmeal, paired with a small amount of protein, can stabilize blood sugar and support restful sleep. Avoiding caffeine and heavy meals late in the evening also aids sleep, allowing the body to recover more effectively overnight.

Understanding Food Sensitivities and Allergies

Food sensitivities can worsen fibromyalgia symptoms, making it essential to identify any adverse reactions to certain foods. Common triggers include gluten, dairy, and certain preservatives, which can contribute to digestive discomfort and inflammation. An elimination diet, where specific foods are removed and reintroduced, can help reveal sensitivities.

Working with a healthcare professional to confirm allergies or intolerances provides clarity and can improve symptom control. By eliminating triggering foods, many people experience reduced pain and more consistent energy levels, leading to improved quality of life.

Keeping a Food Journal to Track Symptoms

A food journal is a valuable tool for tracking how different foods affect fibromyalgia symptoms. Recording meals and noting any resulting changes in pain, energy, or mood helps identify dietary triggers or beneficial foods. Over time, patterns may emerge, making it easier to refine a personalized diet that minimizes discomfort.

The journal doesn't need to be complex; simply write down each meal and any symptoms within a few hours.

This tracking method can also support discussions with healthcare providers and provide insights into effective dietary adjustments that improve overall health.

Consulting with a Nutritionist or Dietitian

Working with a nutritionist or dietitian can provide personalized dietary guidance for managing fibromyalgia. A professional can recommend anti-inflammatory foods, meal planning tips, and potential supplements that align with individual health needs. They can also help identify food sensitivities and design a balanced eating plan to address specific fibromyalgia symptoms.

Consulting a dietitian ensures dietary changes are safe and effective, as they consider medical history and current treatments. With professional support, individuals can make informed decisions about their diet to experience improved symptom management and better overall health.

Preparing Balanced Meals on a Budget

Preparing balanced meals on a budget can help manage fibromyalgia symptoms without overspending. Plan meals around affordable, nutrient-dense ingredients like beans, lentils, eggs, and seasonal vegetables. These foods offer protein, fiber, and vitamins essential for reducing inflammation and maintaining energy levels.

Opt for bulk purchasing of grains and frozen produce to save money, and consider cooking in large batches to freeze for future meals. With smart planning, nutritious, symptom-supporting meals can be both affordable and easy to prepare, providing long-term benefits for fibromyalgia management.

CHAPTER 4:

Exercise and Physical Activity

The Importance of Regular Physical Activity

Regular physical activity plays a crucial role in managing fibromyalgia by helping to reduce pain, stiffness, and fatigue. Engaging in consistent movement can stimulate endorphin production, which acts as a natural pain reliever and mood enhancer. For those with fibromyalgia, movement can feel daunting at first, but starting with simple, small activities like short walks or gentle stretches can create a positive foundation.

Aside from physical benefits, regular activity can improve sleep quality and reduce stress, both of which are essential for fibromyalgia management. Begin by setting small, achievable goals to make exercise a routine part of your life. With time, these efforts help increase strength, flexibility, and endurance, making it easier to perform daily tasks with less discomfort.

Types of Exercises Suitable for Fibromyalgia: Low-Impact and Gentle Activities

Low-impact exercises are particularly beneficial for fibromyalgia, as they minimize stress on joints and muscles. Walking, swimming, or cycling are excellent choices that keep the body moving without causing intense pain or fatigue. These activities are gentler on muscles and help boost overall fitness without overwhelming the body.

Gentle activities like water aerobics or yoga are also ideal, as the water's buoyancy can reduce pressure on joints while providing resistance. Choose exercises you enjoy to make it easier to stay consistent. Over time, low-impact activities can build strength and resilience, making them sustainable for long-term fibromyalgia management.

Stretching and Flexibility Exercises

Regular stretching helps relieve muscle tension, improve flexibility, and reduce stiffness, which are common challenges for those with fibromyalgia. Start with basic stretches targeting large muscle groups, such as gentle hamstring stretches, shoulder rolls, and seated forward bends. Hold each stretch for 10–30 seconds and breathe deeply.

Incorporating a daily stretching routine, even for a few minutes, can greatly enhance your range of motion and reduce pain over time. You can try stretches in the morning to ease stiffness or after other exercises to cool down. As you build flexibility, stretching will become a powerful tool for pain relief and mobility improvement.

Strength Training Basics for Beginners

Strength training can help strengthen muscles and joints, potentially reducing the pain and instability often experienced with fibromyalgia. Begin with body-weight exercises like wall push-ups, seated leg lifts, or using light resistance bands. Start with minimal resistance and short sessions, focusing on form rather than intensity.

Gradually, you can incorporate light weights as your muscles adapt, ensuring each movement is slow and controlled. Avoid lifting heavy or rapid movements, which can lead to soreness or injury. Strength training builds a strong muscular foundation, ultimately supporting better posture and everyday functionality.

Incorporating Aerobic Activities Safely

Aerobic activities, such as walking or stationary cycling, increase heart rate and improve cardiovascular health, which can reduce fatigue and improve energy levels. For fibromyalgia, start with low-intensity sessions, aiming for just five to ten minutes a few times a week, and gradually increase duration as your body adapts.

Choose comfortable environments—like a park or home workout area—to avoid sensory triggers that might cause discomfort. Keep sessions short and adjust based on energy levels to avoid overexertion. Gradual aerobic conditioning can increase stamina, making daily tasks feel easier and less tiring.

Tips for Staying Motivated

Staying motivated is essential, especially with fibromyalgia, where energy and pain levels fluctuate. Set small, realistic goals and celebrate each achievement, such as completing a short walk or a few minutes of stretching. Tracking progress, no matter how small, reinforces a sense of accomplishment and motivates continued effort.

Finding an exercise buddy or joining a supportive community can also help, as it provides accountability and encouragement. Remind yourself of the positive impact on your health and well-being, as even small efforts contribute significantly over time. Consistency, more than intensity, is the key to successful fibromyalgia management.

The Role of Yoga and Tai Chi

Yoga and tai chi are gentle, low-impact practices that combine movement, balance, and breathing, making them ideal for fibromyalgia relief. Yoga stretches muscles and improves flexibility, while tai chi enhances body awareness and balance. Both practices encourage relaxation, helping reduce pain and stress.

Begin with beginner-level classes or online tutorials focused on gentle sequences. Simple poses like Child's Pose or standing Tai Chi movements can help relax muscles without strain. Practicing regularly enhances mind-body connection, making it easier to listen to your body's needs and manage fibromyalgia symptoms.

How to Start an Exercise Routine

To start an exercise routine, begin by identifying your goals—whether to reduce pain, improve mobility, or increase stamina. Begin with short sessions, such as 5–10 minutes of walking or gentle stretching, and build up slowly based on your comfort level. Tracking these initial activities can help you monitor progress.

As you get accustomed to regular movement, gradually introduce variety, such as alternating between strength, flexibility, and aerobic activities. Consistency is more important than intensity, so focus on making exercise a regular, manageable part of your routine. Starting slow and steady sets you up for long-term success.

Monitoring Energy Levels During Exercise

Monitoring energy levels is crucial to avoid overexertion, which can lead to flare-ups in fibromyalgia symptoms. Rate your energy level on a scale of 1–10 before and after exercising, and adjust accordingly. If you feel extremely fatigued, consider a lighter activity or take extra rest.

Use pacing strategies like the "spoon theory" to manage energy effectively, where each exercise takes a "spoon" of energy, helping you balance activities with available stamina. This mindful approach helps you exercise within your limits, minimizing the risk of post-exercise exhaustion.

Creating a Balanced Weekly Exercise Schedule

A balanced exercise schedule for fibromyalgia management includes a mix of flexibility, strength, and aerobic activities spread throughout the week. For example, start with gentle stretching on Mondays, a light aerobic walk on Wednesdays, and body-weight strength exercises on Fridays. Allow rest days in between for muscle recovery.

Keep sessions short and track how you feel after each one, adjusting as needed. This balanced approach ensures that different aspects of fitness are addressed without overwhelming the body. It also supports gradual improvement and helps create a sustainable exercise habit.

Importance of Warm-Up and Cool-Down

Warming up prepares your body for movement by increasing circulation and gently loosening muscles, while cooling down helps reduce soreness and brings heart rate back to normal. For warm-ups, try slow stretches, leg swings, or gentle walking. After exercising, follow with light stretching to relax muscles.

Taking five minutes for warm-up and cool-down can make a noticeable difference in comfort levels, especially with fibromyalgia. These practices help prevent injuries, reduce post-exercise pain, and improve flexibility. Never skip these essential steps, as they help protect muscles and joints.

Avoiding Common Pitfalls and Injuries

Common pitfalls in fibromyalgia-friendly exercise include overexertion, ignoring pain, and lack of rest days. To avoid these, start with low-intensity activities and pay attention to your body's responses. If you experience pain, adjust or switch to a gentler activity instead of pushing through discomfort.

Take breaks and avoid high-impact exercises that can strain muscles and joints. Gradual progression and pacing are key to prevent injury. Remember, with fibromyalgia, exercising smartly within your capacity leads to better, sustainable results than pushing too hard.

Listening to Your Body: Signs to Stop

Listening to your body is essential to avoid overexertion. If you experience intense pain, dizziness, or shortness of breath, stop exercising immediately. These are signals that your body needs a break and that you may need to try a gentler approach.

Fatigue that lasts more than a day after exercise suggests overexertion; in this case, reduce intensity next time. Practicing mindful awareness helps you distinguish between healthy muscle strain and harmful pain, allowing you to adapt workouts safely. This approach helps prevent flare-ups and supports gradual, sustainable progress.

CHAPTER 5:

Sleep and Rest

Importance of Sleep for Fibromyalgia Management

Sleep is vital for managing fibromyalgia symptoms, as restful sleep helps reduce pain and fatigue. Consistent quality sleep can improve mood and mental clarity, both of which are commonly impacted by fibromyalgia. To enhance sleep, focus on maintaining a regular schedule and sleep routine, which can support your body's natural rhythms.

Fibromyalgia patients often experience disrupted sleep cycles, leading to unrefreshed mornings and heightened pain sensitivity. Prioritizing sleep as a key part of fibromyalgia self-care can help mitigate these effects. Establishing a consistent bedtime and wake time helps anchor the body's internal clock, making restful sleep more attainable.

Understanding Sleep Disturbances Related to Fibromyalgia

Fibromyalgia often disrupts sleep through increased wakefulness and issues like non-restorative sleep, where people wake up feeling tired despite long hours in bed. Recognizing these disturbances can help you implement effective sleep strategies tailored to the condition.

Understanding the unique sleep issues associated with fibromyalgia allows you to address underlying factors like anxiety or discomfort. Regularly tracking sleep patterns and recognizing triggers that worsen disturbances can also aid in developing a more effective, individualized approach to restful sleep.

Creating a Sleep-Conducive Environment

To promote restful sleep, create a relaxing sleep environment. Keep the bedroom cool, quiet, and dark; consider using blackout curtains and white noise machines to block disturbances. Invest in a comfortable mattress and pillows that support pain relief.

Minimizing blue light exposure from screens an hour before bed can help improve sleep quality, as blue light interferes with melatonin production. Removing work-related items and electronics from the bedroom can also reinforce that this space is dedicated to relaxation and sleep.

Establishing a Bedtime Routine

A calming bedtime routine signals to your body that it's time to wind down. Gentle stretching, warm baths, and relaxing activities like reading or journaling can ease stress and prepare you for sleep.

Consistently following the same routine helps reinforce these cues for relaxation. Avoid stimulating activities before bed, such as intense conversations or vigorous exercise, to help your body naturally transition to sleep.

Relaxation Techniques for Better Sleep

Relaxation techniques such as deep breathing, progressive muscle relaxation, and guided meditation can help ease the body into sleep. Practicing these techniques regularly makes it easier to unwind, even during flare-ups.

Visualizing calming scenes or focusing on slow, controlled breaths reduces tension, especially helpful for fibromyalgia patients who experience high levels of physical and emotional stress. These methods are easy to practice and can be customized to your preferences for better sleep results.

The Impact of Caffeine and Alcohol on Sleep

Both caffeine and alcohol can disrupt your sleep quality. Caffeine, even in small amounts, can stimulate the nervous system and interfere with falling asleep, while alcohol may make you feel sleepy initially but can fragment your sleep later.

Limit caffeine intake, especially in the afternoon and evening, and consider avoiding alcohol close to bedtime. Reducing reliance on these substances can support your efforts toward a consistent sleep routine, helping to alleviate fibromyalgia symptoms.

Utilizing Sleep Aids and Melatonin

Melatonin supplements can be effective in helping regulate your sleep-wake cycle, especially if you have trouble falling asleep. Start with a low dose to determine what works best, and avoid taking it too close to morning hours to prevent grogginess.

Some over-the-counter sleep aids may also help, but use them sparingly and consult a doctor to prevent dependency or negative interactions with other medications. Always follow recommended dosages and avoid taking aids for extended periods unless prescribed by a healthcare professional.

Napping: When and How Long to Nap Effectively

For fibromyalgia patients, short naps (20-30 minutes) during the afternoon can help recharge without disrupting nighttime sleep. A quick nap can alleviate daytime fatigue but avoid sleeping too long to prevent grogginess.

Establish a consistent napping routine and try to nap in a dark, quiet room for the best results. Longer naps can disrupt nighttime sleep and should be avoided unless needed for extreme fatigue management.

Strategies for Waking Up Refreshed

To wake up feeling more refreshed, expose yourself to natural light in the morning. Sunlight exposure helps reset your internal clock, making it easier to feel alert and awake.

A gentle alarm or gradual wake-up light can reduce the groggy feeling that fibromyalgia patients often experience upon waking. Doing light stretches in bed or slowly moving your muscles can also help ease morning stiffness and prepare you for the day.

Understanding Sleep Cycles

Sleep cycles are crucial in determining the quality of your rest, as each cycle includes light, deep, and REM sleep stages, all essential for restoration. Understanding your cycles helps in optimizing sleep length and avoiding waking up mid-cycle, which can cause grogginess.

Tracking your sleep can give you insights into your sleep stages and allow you to adjust bedtime for a full cycle, making you feel more rested. Apps or devices that monitor sleep can be particularly helpful in understanding your unique patterns.

Managing Restless Leg Syndrome

Restless Leg Syndrome (RLS) can disrupt sleep with an urge to move your legs, often felt as a tingling sensation. Light stretching before bed, warm baths, and magnesium supplements can help reduce RLS symptoms.

Avoiding stimulants and practicing relaxation techniques can also decrease the severity of RLS. Consult a healthcare provider if RLS symptoms persist, as prescription medications are available to manage severe cases.

Keeping a Sleep Diary for Patterns

A sleep diary helps track sleep patterns, which is useful for identifying habits or triggers that interfere with sleep. Note bedtimes, wake times, naps, and factors like diet or stress levels for a full picture.

By analyzing trends in your sleep diary, you can make informed adjustments to your routine. Reviewing this log with your healthcare provider can also help in identifying underlying sleep issues that may need professional attention.

Seeking Medical Advice for Sleep Issues

If sleep issues persist despite lifestyle changes, consult a healthcare provider who can assess for sleep disorders commonly associated with fibromyalgia, such as sleep apnea or insomnia. A sleep study may be recommended to evaluate your sleep quality.

Medical advice is valuable for chronic sleep issues, as tailored therapies or treatments, including cognitive behavioral therapy for insomnia (CBT-I), can improve sleep over time. Early intervention may prevent further sleep complications and alleviate fibromyalgia symptoms effectively.

CHAPTER 6:

Stress Management Techniques

Understanding the Link between Stress and Fibromyalgia

Stress is a significant factor that can worsen fibromyalgia symptoms, as it triggers the body's pain response, heightening sensitivity and fatigue. Recognizing how stress interacts with fibromyalgia allows individuals to proactively manage it, potentially reducing pain and improving quality of life. Studies indicate that the nervous system becomes more reactive in fibromyalgia patients, making stress management critical for alleviating symptoms.

Managing stress can reduce pain levels and increase resilience against flare-ups. Simple daily habits, like setting aside time for self-care or engaging in relaxing activities, can help stabilize the nervous system. Understanding this connection encourages individuals to adopt practices to counteract stress's effects, such as meditation, exercise, or structured relaxation techniques.

Techniques for Identifying Stress Triggers

Identifying stress triggers is crucial in managing fibromyalgia as certain situations can unknowingly intensify symptoms. Common triggers might include workplace deadlines, social obligations, or even household tasks. Keeping a daily journal to record situations, emotions, and symptom changes helps identify specific triggers, revealing patterns that increase stress.

Once recognized, triggers can be mitigated with preemptive steps such as delegating tasks, adjusting schedules, or planning breaks. The awareness that comes from identifying these triggers allows for targeted strategies to reduce stress impact, improving overall well-being and helping manage fibromyalgia symptoms more effectively.

Deep Breathing Exercises and Their Benefits

Deep breathing exercises can help relax the nervous system, reducing fibromyalgia-related tension and stress. Simple techniques, such as the 4-7-8 method (inhale for 4 seconds, hold for 7, exhale for 8), help regulate heart rate and promote a calm state. Practicing this daily or during stressful moments provides immediate relaxation benefits, supporting both mental and physical health.

These exercises are easily incorporated into routines—whether sitting at a desk, lying down, or during a break. Regular deep breathing can reduce pain perception and boost energy by supplying oxygen to muscles, relieving tightness, and promoting relaxation that is beneficial for fibromyalgia sufferers.

Mindfulness and Meditation Practices

Mindfulness meditation helps people focus on the present moment, reducing stress and enhancing emotional control, which is especially helpful for managing fibromyalgia. Starting with a simple practice—like sitting quietly and focusing on breathing for five minutes daily—can make a noticeable difference. Observing thoughts without judgment encourages a calm mental state, reducing the anxiety that often accompanies chronic pain.

Guided meditations, which can be accessed through apps, offer structured ways to relax and disengage from stressful thoughts. Regular mindfulness practice can also reduce pain intensity, as studies show it decreases reactivity to pain signals in the brain, providing a sense of control over fibromyalgia symptoms.

Progressive Muscle Relaxation Techniques

Progressive muscle relaxation (PMR) is an effective way to relieve muscle tension commonly associated with fibromyalgia. This technique involves tensing each muscle group for a few seconds and then releasing, starting from the toes and moving upwards. PMR sessions can last 10-15 minutes and are best done lying down in a quiet space.

By focusing on releasing tension systematically, PMR can reduce stress and alleviate physical discomfort. Over time, PMR enhances body awareness and control, making it easier to recognize and manage tension that can exacerbate fibromyalgia pain.

The Importance of Time Management

Good time management helps prevent the overwhelm that can trigger fibromyalgia symptoms. Prioritizing tasks and setting realistic goals for each day can make a significant difference. Using tools like planners or digital apps, individuals can organize activities, allowing for breaks and focusing on one thing at a time.

Time management includes allotting time for self-care, ensuring rest periods, and balancing work and personal life. By managing time effectively, individuals avoid over-exertion and reduce the risk of stress-induced flare-ups, supporting better symptom control.

Setting Boundaries in Personal and Professional Life

Setting boundaries in relationships and at work is essential to avoid stress that may worsen fibromyalgia symptoms. Clear communication about limits—whether it's saying "no" to extra responsibilities or expressing needs to loved ones—helps conserve energy and reduce tension. Begin by identifying where you feel overwhelmed and practice assertive communication.

Establishing these boundaries allows individuals to protect their energy and focus on wellness, a practice that supports consistent symptom management.

Boundaries create a buffer from stress, helping maintain balance and reducing fibromyalgia flares caused by physical and emotional overextension.

Finding Hobbies and Interests for Stress Relief

Engaging in hobbies and activities is a powerful way to relieve stress and distract from fibromyalgia discomfort. Choose activities that align with personal interests and require minimal physical strain, like painting, gardening, or listening to music. Such hobbies encourage relaxation and create opportunities to disconnect from stressors.

Creative outlets also offer an emotional release, contributing to mental well-being. Even short daily sessions spent on a favorite hobby provide stress relief, emotional enrichment, and positive distractions from pain, ultimately supporting a healthier lifestyle for managing fibromyalgia.

The Benefits of Laughter and Socializing

Laughter and social interaction naturally reduce stress, releasing endorphins that improve mood and decrease pain perception. Watching a comedy, spending time with friends, or attending social events in moderation can provide much-needed joy and relaxation. For fibromyalgia sufferers, laughter offers a lighthearted way to break from the cycle of pain and fatigue.

Socializing, even in small amounts, nurtures a sense of connection and combats isolation often associated with chronic pain. These interactions can be tailored to energy levels, such as virtual meet-ups or brief gatherings, to maintain a supportive network without exhausting oneself.

Support Groups and Their Importance

Support groups provide an understanding environment for individuals with fibromyalgia to share experiences and gain insights. Being part of a community that understands similar challenges reduces feelings of isolation and provides valuable coping strategies. Many groups meet virtually, offering flexibility for those managing fluctuating energy levels.

These connections can also lead to discovering new approaches to symptom management. Support groups offer emotional encouragement and practical advice, making the journey of managing fibromyalgia less overwhelming and more supported.

Utilizing Journaling for Emotional Processing

Journaling provides a private space to express emotions, track symptoms, and reflect on daily challenges. Writing about stressors, pain experiences, or even gratitude helps release emotions and provides clarity on stress patterns. By noting down feelings and experiences, individuals can identify triggers and coping strategies that work.

Over time, journaling can become a therapeutic practice that improves self-awareness and emotional regulation, which are crucial for fibromyalgia management. It's also an effective way to track progress, celebrate small wins, and understand what brings relief or exacerbates symptoms.

The Role of Pets and Nature in Stress Reduction

Interacting with pets and spending time in nature have shown significant benefits in reducing stress and improving mood. Pets provide companionship, which eases loneliness, while their calming presence has been proven to lower stress hormones. Walking a pet or spending time with animals can promote light exercise, beneficial for muscle stiffness and mental clarity.

Likewise, spending time outdoors offers fresh air, sunlight, and a calming environment that aids relaxation. Nature activities like short walks, gardening, or even sitting in a park can improve mood and provide a comforting break from the routine, supporting better mental and physical health.

Professional Help: When to Seek Counseling

Seeking counseling can be an essential part of managing fibromyalgia, especially if stress or emotional distress becomes overwhelming. Therapists trained in cognitive-behavioral therapy (CBT) can help individuals develop tools for managing pain and stress, including techniques for reinterpreting pain perception and strengthening resilience.

Counseling provides a safe space to explore complex emotions linked to chronic pain, such as frustration or grief. For fibromyalgia sufferers, professional guidance supports emotional health and offers coping strategies tailored to personal needs, which can significantly improve overall quality of life.

CHAPTER 7

Building a Support System

Importance of Having a Support Network

Building a strong support network is crucial for managing fibromyalgia, as it provides emotional and practical assistance. Friends, family, and peers who understand your condition can offer encouragement and empathy, reducing feelings of isolation. This network can also help you navigate daily challenges, making it easier to cope with symptoms and maintain a positive outlook.

To establish a support network, start by reaching out to loved ones and sharing your experiences with fibromyalgia. Let them know how they can help, whether it's by accompanying you to appointments or simply being there to listen. Consider engaging with others in your community who understand your situation, as they can provide valuable insights and reassurance.

Educating Family and Friends about Fibromyalgia

Educating your family and friends about fibromyalgia is essential for fostering understanding and support. Begin by explaining what fibromyalgia is, its symptoms, and how it affects your daily life. Use simple language and relatable examples to convey your experiences, emphasizing that it is a real condition that can significantly impact your well-being.

Encourage your loved ones to ask questions and engage in conversations about fibromyalgia. Providing them with resources, such as articles or videos, can help deepen their understanding. This knowledge will enable them to be more compassionate and supportive, making it easier for you to share your journey with them.

Finding Local or Online Support Groups

Finding local or online support groups can be an invaluable resource for individuals with fibromyalgia. These groups offer a safe space to share experiences, exchange advice, and receive emotional support from others who understand your struggles. Start by researching local community centers, hospitals, or health organizations that may host support groups.

For online options, search social media platforms or websites dedicated to chronic pain and fibromyalgia. Joining forums or discussion groups can provide instant access to a wealth of knowledge and shared experiences. These connections can significantly enhance your emotional resilience and provide practical tips for managing your condition.

How to Communicate Your Needs Effectively

Effectively communicating your needs is vital for managing fibromyalgia. Start by being clear and assertive about your symptoms and limitations. Use "I" statements to express how fibromyalgia affects you, such as, "I feel fatigued after long periods of activity," which helps others understand your perspective without feeling defensive.

Practice open dialogue with your support network, allowing them to ask questions and share their thoughts. This two-way communication fosters empathy and ensures that your needs are recognized and accommodated, ultimately enhancing your relationships and support system.

The Role of Advocacy in Self-Care

Advocacy plays a critical role in self-care for fibromyalgia sufferers. By advocating for yourself, you can ensure that your healthcare providers understand your condition and are responsive to your needs. Start by educating yourself about fibromyalgia and the latest treatment options, which empowers you to speak confidently about your care.

You can also advocate for fibromyalgia awareness in your community by participating in local events or sharing your experiences online. By raising awareness, you not only support your journey but also help others understand and empathize with the condition, creating a more supportive environment for everyone affected.

Seeking Help from Healthcare Professionals

Seeking help from healthcare professionals is essential for effective fibromyalgia management. Start by identifying a healthcare provider familiar with fibromyalgia, such as a rheumatologist or pain specialist. Schedule an appointment to discuss your symptoms and explore tailored treatment options, which may include medication, physical therapy, or alternative therapies.

Be open and honest about your experiences during your appointments, providing specific details about your symptoms and their impact on your life. Collaborating with your healthcare provider helps develop a comprehensive treatment plan that addresses your unique needs and improves your quality of life.

Connecting with Other Patients for Shared Experiences

Connecting with other patients who have fibromyalgia can be incredibly beneficial for sharing experiences and coping strategies. You can find these connections through support groups, online forums, or social media platforms. Engaging in conversations with those who understand your struggles can provide comfort, validation, and valuable insights into managing your condition.

Consider attending meetups or virtual gatherings to deepen these connections. Sharing stories and discussing challenges can foster a sense of belonging and inspire new approaches to managing symptoms, ultimately enhancing your emotional well-being.

Importance of Community Resources

Utilizing community resources is crucial for enhancing your self-care plan in managing fibromyalgia. Local health departments, community centers, and non-profit organizations often provide resources such as counseling services, fitness classes, or educational workshops tailored to chronic pain management. Start by researching what resources are available in your area.

Take advantage of these offerings to gain new skills, build social connections, and access support. Engaging with community resources can help reduce isolation and provide opportunities for personal growth, ultimately contributing to your overall well-being.

Discussing Financial Assistance Options

Discussing financial assistance options can ease the burden of managing fibromyalgia-related costs. Start by researching local and national organizations that offer grants, scholarships, or financial aid specifically for individuals with chronic conditions. Some healthcare providers also have financial counselors who can help navigate insurance options and payment plans.

Don't hesitate to reach out to non-profit organizations focused on fibromyalgia, as they may have resources and support systems in place. By exploring these options, you can reduce financial stress and focus more on your health and well-being.

Utilizing Social Media for Support and Information

Social media can be a powerful tool for finding support and information about fibromyalgia. Join groups or follow pages dedicated to fibromyalgia awareness, where members share experiences, coping strategies, and valuable resources. Engaging in these online communities allows you to connect with others who understand your journey and can offer support.

Additionally, use social media to stay informed about the latest research, treatment options, and events related to fibromyalgia. By following credible sources and advocates, you can enhance your understanding of the condition and empower yourself to make informed decisions about your care.

Engaging in Group Activities or Classes

Participating in group activities or classes can enhance your well-being and help manage fibromyalgia symptoms. Look for local classes, such as yoga, tai chi, or art therapy, that focus on gentle movement and relaxation techniques. These activities not only promote physical health but also provide social interactions that can improve mood and reduce feelings of isolation.

To get started, check local community centers, fitness studios, or online platforms offering virtual classes. By engaging in group activities, you can learn new skills, build connections, and find joy in shared experiences while effectively managing your symptoms.

The Benefits of Volunteering and Giving Back

Volunteering can be a rewarding way to cope with fibromyalgia while positively impacting your community. Engaging in volunteer work can provide a sense of purpose and fulfillment, which is vital for emotional well-being. Start by identifying causes that resonate with you and look for local organizations that align with your interests.

Even small acts of service can make a difference. Choose tasks that fit your energy levels and schedule, allowing you to contribute without overexerting yourself. By giving back, you can foster connections, create a support network, and enhance your overall quality of life.

Celebrating Small Victories with Your Support Network

Celebrating small victories with your support network is essential for maintaining motivation and a positive mindset. Recognize and acknowledge achievements, whether it's managing a challenging day or sticking to a self-care routine. Sharing these milestones with your loved ones creates a sense of shared joy and encouragement.

Consider setting aside time to reflect on your progress, perhaps through a small gathering or an online chat. This practice not only reinforces your commitment to self-care but also strengthens the bonds within your support network, fostering a sense of community and shared understanding.

CHAPTER 8:

Tracking Progress and Adjusting Your Plan

Importance of Tracking Symptoms and Triggers

Tracking symptoms and triggers is essential for managing fibromyalgia effectively. By documenting daily experiences, individuals can identify patterns in their pain, fatigue, and other symptoms, helping them understand what exacerbates or alleviates their condition. This information is crucial for making informed decisions about self-care and treatment options.

To get started, consider creating a simple chart or using a notebook to note the severity of symptoms, activities engaged in, and emotional states. By maintaining consistency in tracking, patterns may emerge over time, revealing specific triggers such as certain foods, stressors, or physical activities. This awareness enables more tailored self-care strategies.

Keeping a Comprehensive Health Journal

A health journal serves as a valuable tool in managing fibromyalgia symptoms. Documenting daily symptoms, treatments, medications, and emotional well-being allows for a holistic view of one's health. This journal can become a reference point for discussions with healthcare providers, ensuring that nothing important is overlooked during appointments.

To create an effective health journal, dedicate a section to each category, such as pain levels, fatigue, diet, and emotional state. This organized approach makes it easier to spot trends and correlations, enabling better self-management strategies. Regularly updating the journal ensures that it remains a current and helpful resource.

Evaluating the Effectiveness of Treatments

Regular evaluation of treatments is vital for effective fibromyalgia management. Understanding which therapies and medications provide relief can inform future decisions about self-care strategies. Keeping track of how symptoms respond to various treatments helps refine approaches to care, maximizing relief and minimizing unnecessary side effects.

To assess treatment effectiveness, maintain a list of medications and therapies, noting changes in symptoms over time. This can include documenting any side effects or improvements experienced. By reviewing this information regularly, individuals can have informed conversations with healthcare providers about possible adjustments to their treatment plan.

Setting Realistic Goals for Symptom Management

Setting realistic goals is crucial for managing fibromyalgia symptoms without feeling overwhelmed. By establishing achievable objectives, individuals can create a structured approach to self-care that enhances motivation and provides a sense of accomplishment. Goals may include simple tasks, such as walking for 10 minutes each day or trying a new relaxation technique weekly.

When setting goals, focus on the SMART criteria: Specific, Measurable, Achievable, Relevant, and Time-bound. For example, instead of a vague goal like "exercise more," specify "walk for 15 minutes three times a week." This clarity not only enhances focus but also fosters a greater sense of control over one's health journey.

Understanding When to Adjust Self-Care Strategies

Self-care strategies must evolve as symptoms and triggers change over time. Recognizing when it's time to adjust these strategies is critical to ongoing symptom management. Monitoring how effective current practices are helps identify when to seek new techniques or therapies, ensuring that care remains responsive to changing needs.

To determine if a strategy needs adjustment, regularly assess symptom patterns and overall well-being. If specific activities or treatments no longer provide relief or seem to exacerbate symptoms, it's time to explore alternative options. Consulting with healthcare providers can also help identify new approaches tailored to current health needs.

Communicating Changes with Healthcare Providers

Effective communication with healthcare providers is essential for managing fibromyalgia. Sharing updates about symptoms, triggers, and the effectiveness of treatments can lead to better care decisions and support. Clear communication ensures that healthcare providers have a complete picture of an individual's health, enabling them to recommend appropriate adjustments.

To facilitate communication, consider preparing for appointments by summarizing key changes in a health journal. Bring specific examples of symptom changes or responses to treatments. This proactive approach helps healthcare providers tailor their recommendations to fit individual circumstances, improving overall management strategies.

The Role of Technology in Tracking Health Data

Technology plays a pivotal role in tracking health data for individuals managing fibromyalgia. Many apps and digital platforms allow users to log symptoms, medications, and other health-related information easily. This convenience enables more accurate tracking and can provide insights that may be overlooked in traditional methods.

To utilize technology effectively, explore various health tracking apps designed for chronic pain management. Look for features such as symptom logging, medication reminders, and mood tracking. These tools can simplify the process of monitoring health and provide valuable data for discussions with healthcare providers, enhancing overall management.

Utilizing Apps or Charts for Symptom Tracking

Using apps or charts for symptom tracking can significantly enhance fibromyalgia management. These tools simplify the process of documenting symptoms, allowing for easy visualization of patterns over time. By regularly inputting data, individuals can identify triggers and effective coping strategies, facilitating better self-management.

To get started, select an app or create a simple chart that includes categories such as pain levels, fatigue, sleep quality, and emotional well-being. Regularly updating this information helps build a comprehensive picture of health. Many apps also offer reminders and analysis features, making it easier to stay engaged with self-care.

Assessing Emotional Well-Being

Emotional well-being is a critical aspect of managing fibromyalgia, as chronic pain cans significantly impact mental health. Regularly assessing feelings and emotional states can provide insights into how well individuals are coping with their condition. This awareness allows for the identification of when additional support or adjustments to self-care strategies may be necessary.

To assess emotional well-being, consider keeping a section in a health journal dedicated to feelings and mood fluctuations. Engaging in self-reflection through journaling or guided practices can help articulate emotions and highlight patterns related to pain and fatigue. If negative emotions persist, seeking professional support from a counselor or therapist may be beneficial.

Regularly Reviewing Dietary Habits

Diet can significantly influence fibromyalgia symptoms, making regular review of dietary habits essential. Understanding how different foods affect energy levels, pain, and overall health can guide individuals in making healthier choices that support their well-being. Identifying food triggers helps create a personalized dietary plan that can alleviate symptoms.

To review dietary habits effectively, keep a food diary that tracks meals and any corresponding symptoms. This practice helps identify patterns, such as increased pain after consuming certain foods. Consulting a registered dietitian familiar with fibromyalgia can provide additional guidance on creating a balanced, anti-inflammatory diet that supports overall health.

Importance of Flexibility in Your Care Plan

Flexibility in a self-care plan is vital for effectively managing fibromyalgia symptoms. Since symptoms can fluctuate, being open to adjusting approaches allows individuals to respond to changing needs without frustration. A rigid plan may lead to disappointment if expectations aren't met, while flexibility promotes resilience and adaptability.

To cultivate flexibility, approach self-care with an open mind. If a particular strategy isn't working, be willing to try something new or modify existing routines. Regularly evaluate the effectiveness of various practices and adjust them based on current symptoms, maintaining a focus on self-compassion and personal well-being.

Celebrating Progress, No Matter How Small

Celebrating progress, no matter how small, is crucial for maintaining motivation in managing fibromyalgia. Acknowledging achievements—such as reducing pain, improving sleep quality, or completing self-care tasks—can foster a positive mindset and reinforce commitment to self-care. Celebrating these milestones cultivates a sense of empowerment.

To celebrate progress, consider keeping a "success journal" where you document achievements and positive changes. Share these victories with supportive friends or family members to enhance the celebration. By focusing on progress, individuals can stay motivated and resilient in their journey toward better health.

Learning from Setbacks and Moving Forward

Setbacks are a natural part of managing fibromyalgia, and learning from them can lead to personal growth. Rather than viewing setbacks as failures, approach them as opportunities to reflect on what may have contributed to a flare-up or change in symptoms. This mindset fosters resilience and helps refine self-care strategies moving forward.

To learn from setbacks, take time to analyze what may have led to a decline in well-being. Consider documenting these reflections in a journal and identifying what changes can be made to avoid similar situations in the future. By focusing on growth and adaptability, individuals can continue to progress despite challenges.

CHAPTER 9:

Frequently Asked Questions (FAQs)

What is the best treatment for fibromyalgia?

The best treatment for fibromyalgia often involves a combination of medication, therapy, and lifestyle changes tailored to the individual's symptoms. Medications may include pain relievers, antidepressants, and anti-seizure drugs, which can help manage pain and improve sleep quality. In addition, cognitive behavioral therapy (CBT) is effective for addressing emotional and psychological challenges associated with chronic pain.

To find the most effective treatment, it's essential to work closely with a healthcare provider who understands fibromyalgia. This collaboration allows for regular adjustments to the treatment plan based on symptom changes and responses to various therapies, ensuring the approach remains effective over time.

How can I improve my quality of life with fibromyalgia?

Improving quality of life with fibromyalgia involves establishing a consistent daily routine that prioritizes self-care. This includes regular sleep patterns, nutritious meals, and scheduled physical activity. Engaging in relaxing activities, such as yoga or meditation, can also help alleviate stress and promote mental well-being, which is crucial in managing symptoms.

Additionally, keeping a symptom diary can help identify triggers and patterns in pain, fatigue, or mood changes. By recognizing these factors, you can make informed decisions about your daily activities and lifestyle choices, further enhancing your overall well-being.

Are there any specific diets that help with fibromyalgia?

While there is no one-size-fits-all diet for fibromyalgia, many people find relief by adopting an anti-inflammatory diet. This typically includes whole foods, such as fruits, vegetables, whole grains, and lean proteins, while avoiding processed foods, sugars, and trans fats. Incorporating omega-3 fatty acids found in fish and flaxseed can also reduce inflammation and promote better health.

Experimenting with food sensitivities is another practical step. Many individuals report symptom improvement by eliminating common allergens like gluten or dairy from their diets. Keeping a food diary can help track changes in symptoms related to dietary modifications, allowing you to identify which foods may help or hinder your condition.

How can I manage fibromyalgia while working?

Managing fibromyalgia while working requires open communication with your employer and flexibility in your work environment. Consider discussing accommodations that can reduce physical strain, such as adjustable desks or flexible hours to accommodate fatigue. Prioritizing tasks and breaking them into manageable steps can also help prevent overwhelm and maintain productivity.

Additionally, practicing good self-care during work hours is crucial. Taking regular breaks to stretch, practice deep breathing, or engage in brief physical activity can help manage pain and fatigue. Finding a supportive colleague or mentor to share your experiences with can also provide emotional relief and foster understanding in the workplace.

What are the best exercises for fibromyalgia?

The best exercises for fibromyalgia are low-impact activities that promote flexibility, strength, and cardiovascular health. Walking, swimming, and cycling are excellent options, as they are gentle on the joints while providing essential physical benefits. Aim for 30 minutes of exercise most days of the week, starting with shorter sessions and gradually increasing duration as tolerated.

Incorporating stretching and relaxation exercises like yoga or tai chi can also significantly help in managing symptoms. These practices improve flexibility and reduce stress, which can lead to decreased pain levels and improved overall well-being. Always listen to your body and consult a healthcare professional before starting a new exercise regimen.

How do I talk to my doctor about my symptoms?

When discussing your symptoms with a doctor, it's helpful to prepare a detailed account of your experiences. Keep a symptom diary that records when symptoms occur, their severity, and any potential triggers. This documentation provides a clear picture of your condition, allowing the doctor to make more informed decisions regarding your treatment options.

Be honest and open about how your symptoms affect your daily life, including work, relationships, and emotional well-being. Asking specific questions about potential treatments or management strategies can facilitate a more productive conversation and empower you to take an active role in your care.

Is fibromyalgia a progressive disease?

Fibromyalgia is not considered a progressive disease, meaning it does not typically worsen over time in a predictable way like some other chronic conditions. However, symptoms can fluctuate, leading to periods of increased pain or fatigue, often referred to as "flares." Understanding this variability can help you manage expectations and prepare for changes in symptom intensity.

It's crucial to focus on effective management strategies rather than worrying about progression. With appropriate treatment, many individuals successfully manage their symptoms and lead fulfilling lives. Staying proactive about health and wellness can help maintain stability and improve long-term quality of life.

Can fibromyalgia be cured?

Currently, there is no known cure for fibromyalgia, but many individuals find ways to effectively manage their symptoms and improve their quality of life. Treatment plans typically focus on alleviating pain, reducing fatigue, and addressing associated mental health issues. Through a combination of medication, therapy, and lifestyle changes, many people experience significant symptom relief.

Emphasizing self-care, including regular exercise, a healthy diet, and stress management techniques, can play a critical role in controlling symptoms. By taking a comprehensive approach to management, individuals can often achieve a balance that allows them to live actively and meaningfully despite their diagnosis.

How can I manage flares and increase my energy levels?

Managing flares requires a proactive approach to identify triggers and implement strategies to minimize their impact. Keeping a diary can help you track patterns and recognize potential stressors, allowing for timely adjustments in your routine. During a flare, prioritize rest and self-care, and consider techniques such as gentle stretching, warm baths, or relaxation exercises to alleviate discomfort.

To increase energy levels, focus on maintaining a balanced diet and staying hydrated. Small, frequent meals rich in nutrients can help stabilize energy throughout the day. Additionally, incorporating short bouts of low-impact exercise can enhance stamina and combat fatigue over time, making it easier to manage daily activities during flare-ups.

Are there any alternative therapies that help?

Many individuals with fibromyalgia explore alternative therapies to complement their conventional treatments. Options like acupuncture, massage therapy, and chiropractic care can provide significant relief from pain and promote relaxation. It's essential to seek practitioners experienced in treating chronic pain conditions for the best outcomes.

Mind-body therapies such as mindfulness meditation, guided imagery, and biofeedback can also be beneficial. These practices help individuals develop coping strategies for managing pain and stress, improving overall emotional health. Always consult with a healthcare provider before starting any new therapies to ensure they align with your treatment plan.

How does stress affect fibromyalgia symptoms?

Stress plays a significant role in exacerbating fibromyalgia symptoms. When stressed, the body releases hormones that can intensify pain perception, leading to increased fatigue and discomfort. Identifying stressors and implementing coping strategies can help mitigate their effects, thereby reducing symptom severity.

Effective stress management techniques include deep breathing exercises, mindfulness practices, and engaging in hobbies or activities that bring joy and relaxation. Building a support system of friends, family, or support groups can also provide emotional relief, helping to manage stress and improve overall quality of life.

What should I do if my treatment isn't working?

If your treatment isn't yielding the desired results, it's important to communicate openly with your healthcare provider. They can evaluate your current regimen and consider adjustments, such as changing medications, incorporating new therapies, or exploring alternative approaches. Regular follow-ups are crucial in finding an effective strategy tailored to your needs.

Additionally, consider seeking a second opinion or consulting a specialist in fibromyalgia or chronic pain management. Sometimes, a fresh perspective can uncover new treatment options or strategies you haven't yet tried, enhancing your chances of finding relief from your symptoms.

How can I find a good support group?

Finding a good support group for fibromyalgia can provide invaluable emotional support and practical advice. Start by researching local community resources, hospitals, or wellness centers that may host support groups. Online platforms like social media or dedicated health forums can also be excellent places to connect with others who share similar experiences.

When looking for a group, consider factors such as the group's size, structure, and focus. Some groups may focus on emotional support, while others might emphasize sharing treatment strategies. Joining a group that aligns with your needs can foster connections and provide a sense of community that is often crucial in managing chronic conditions.

Recap the Importance of a Comprehensive Self-Care Plan

A comprehensive self-care plan is crucial for managing fibromyalgia, as it allows individuals to tailor their approaches based on their unique symptoms and lifestyle. By addressing various aspects such as physical health, emotional well-being, and daily routines, a well-rounded self-care plan provides a structured way to navigate the challenges of chronic pain. Incorporating activities like gentle exercise, mindfulness, and proper nutrition can enhance overall health and mitigate symptoms.

Implementing a self-care plan requires commitment and consistency. It's essential to regularly evaluate what works and what doesn't, making adjustments as needed. Tracking symptoms and progress can help identify patterns, empowering individuals to make informed decisions about their care and enabling them to engage actively in their health journey.

Encourage Continuous Learning and Adaptation

Continuous learning about fibromyalgia and its treatment options is key to effective self-management. Staying informed through reputable sources, attending workshops, or joining support groups can provide valuable insights and strategies that may improve one's condition. It also fosters a sense of community, allowing individuals to share experiences and learn from each other.

Adaptation is equally important as individuals discover what strategies best alleviate their symptoms. By remaining flexible and open to change, one can explore new therapies, lifestyle modifications, or self-care techniques that enhance their quality of life. This mindset not only promotes resilience but also helps in finding what truly works for each person's unique situation.

Empower Individuals to Take Control of Their Health

Taking control of one's health involves actively participating in treatment decisions and self-care practices. This can include collaborating with healthcare providers to create personalized care plans that encompass medication management, physical therapy, and alternative treatments. Understanding the options available empowers individuals to advocate for themselves and make informed choices.

Moreover, engaging in self-education about fibromyalgia can help demystify the condition, reducing feelings of helplessness. By learning to recognize triggers and symptoms, individuals can implement preventative measures and techniques to manage flare-ups effectively, fostering a proactive approach to health and well-being.

Remind Readers That They Are Not Alone in Their Journey

Living with fibromyalgia can feel isolating, but it's essential to remember that support is available. Many individuals share similar experiences, and connecting with others through support groups, forums, or social media can provide comfort and understanding. Sharing stories and coping strategies helps build a sense of community, reminding individuals that they are not facing their struggles alone.

Professional help, such as therapy or counseling, can also play a significant role in combating feelings of isolation. These resources provide a safe space to express emotions and receive guidance, reinforcing the idea that seeking help is a sign of strength and an essential part of the healing process.

Highlight the Potential for Improvement and a Better Quality of Life

While fibromyalgia poses significant challenges, many individuals experience improvements over time with the right strategies in place. By implementing a tailored self-care plan that includes regular exercise, proper nutrition, and stress management techniques, individuals can reduce symptoms and enhance their overall well-being. Small, consistent changes can lead to substantial progress, illustrating that a better quality of life is possible.

It's important to celebrate milestones, no matter how small, as they contribute to a sense of accomplishment and motivation.

www.ingramcontent.com/pod-product-compliance
Lightning Source LLC
Chambersburg PA
CBHW061650250726
48659CB00004B/1448